THE GRASS
IS GREENER
WHEN
THE SUN
IS YELLOW

SARAH ROSENTHAL
&
VALERIE WITTE

the operating system print//document

THE GRASS IS GREENER WHEN THE SUN IS YELLOW

ISBN # 978-1-946031-67-9
copyright © 2019 by Sarah Rosenthal and Valerie Witte
edited and designed by ELÆ [Lynne DeSilva-Johnson]

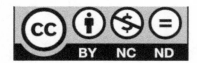

For additional questions regarding reproduction, quotation, or to request a pdf for review contact operator@theoperatingsystem.org

Print books from The Operating System are distributed to the trade via Ingram, with additional production by Spencer Printing, in Honesdale, PA, in the USA. Digital books are available directly from the OS, direct from authors, via DIY pamplet printing, and/or POD.

This text was set in Steelworks Vintage, Europa-Light, Minion, and OCR-A Standard.

Cover Art uses an image from the series "Collected Objects & the Dead Birds I Did Not Carry Home," by Heidi Reszies.

the operating system
www.theoperatingsystem.org
mailto: operator@theoperatingsystem.org

THE GRASS
IS GREENER
WHEN
THE SUN
IS YELLOW

For

Simone Forti

and

Yvonne Rainer

POETS' NOTE

We launched our collaboration by reading and discussing *Eternal Apprentice,* a chapbook by Michael Newton and Emmalea Russo (DoubleCross, 2016) in which the authors converse with each other about the book-making process. As part of their discussion, they engage with John Cage and Merce Cunningham's ideas about chance operations. We became interested in using the chapbook as a source text, as well as in employing random procedures in our project.

In addition, we noted Cunningham's role as a key figure in the evolution of contemporary dance, influencing several female choreographers who went on to make significant contributions to the field. We also discovered that the two of us had radically different feelings about dance: Sarah has a mostly positive relationship to the form, having engaged with dance in various contexts throughout her life, whereas dance has more troublesome associations for Valerie, bringing up feelings of insecurity and deficiency. We decided to each "adopt" a contemporary female dancer-choreographer who had worked at some point with Cunningham and Cage, letting our contributions be informed and inspired by these innovative women's lives and ideas, and thinking through our own respective relationships to dance. Valerie chose Simone Forti and Sarah chose Yvonne Rainer.

We created a series of sonnets, lifting lines from the chapbook to serve as the first line of each sonnet. Poet A emailed a first line to Poet B, who replied with a second line plus a theme for the poem. We continued trading lines until we reached the requisite 14; we had several sonnets under construction at once. Italicized language in the sonnets is lifted or adapted from various texts and works by and about Forti and Rainer.

The poems are interwoven with letters we wrote to each other, musing on the sonnets and allowing ourselves to be carried by association and the call-and-response nature of epistolary form into the exploration of various arcs and tangents.

In developing this project's contours, we relied on our curiosity and a desire to take creative risks. Yet looking back, we recognize the shared feminist tenets that undergird this work. Collaborating on the poems' composition (and incorporating the work and words of Rainer and Forti, who in a sense become additional collaborators) challenges the traditional Western concept of the text written by a solo (male) author.

The epistolary component, in which we give ourselves the luxury of asking and answering questions about our contributions to the poems, adds embodiment to a project highly mediated by technology. In the letters we "show our hand" to one another and to the reader, creating a space of intimacy and vulnerability. Yet we strive to do so in a way that opens up, rather than forecloses, multiple readings of the poems. Each of us, and by extension our readers, are invited to "talk back" and bring other perspectives to the conversation. We strive to construct an environment that is both challenging and invitational, because that's the world we want to live, learn, and create in.

TABLE OF CONTENTS

eyelids inscribed with your dream

what is an eyelid *open as a window / I miss the trees*

filmic I wake to your tattoo / open window

made or shamed me but I could never be / choreographed

breath and REM the rhythm that moved me

in waves as shapes / awaken my dormant limbs

to carve the space of missing / trees

or the negative we inhabit but is it / still / a story

a *no to virtuosity*

a wanting to be seen or held in regard / in / visible

stripped / available

as if leaning no lying / down

your dream tattooed on my sleeping frame

<u>we are advised to start fresh</u>

then he tells me my name; shall I call this practice?

entering and uttering and

huddling through my motor centers

replace names with games / arrive at a practice

if I wanted to play but boys never need to know how

if I gave numbers to my motor centers

for one night tried only to stand / *and I was in one of the boxes*

repeating *the grass is / greener when the sun / is yellow*

longing for *roots of dance / what I knew about things through my body*

the feeling I had when I ran

no longer a girl / *stilled*

the stage lights fade up / I face them

am I ready for my curtain call?

Dear Valerie,

Thanks for being open to folding letters into our already elaborate collaborative plan! Since we don't know each other very well, this might help us sense the embodied beings behind lines arriving out of the ether. I'll dive right in with thoughts on our first poem, "I have always wanted to film myself sleeping." I was puzzled by the first line/title, which you provided, and to be honest, initially felt resistant to it—confronted by the challenge of inhabiting an "I" that I'd never encountered or imagined before. Ultimately I developed a relationship with the line through an association I had to a film by Lynn Hershman. The film includes a repeating image of a naked woman lying on the crest of a sand dune, then rolling down it. I was also thinking about dreams (because I'm always thinking about dreams). I addressed my response line to a "you" which I thought of as you-the-film-audience and you-the-reader as well as other possible "you's." "Inscribed" adds the sense of writing as a sensual act, a kind of body henna or tattoo.

I kept the film and inscription ideas in my next line. I liked the ideas I found in your line both of the eyelid as a kind of window and of eyes opening and the gaze landing, first thing, on a window. I was intrigued by your slash and wanted to try it out. Your next line made me think of Yvonne Rainer and other experimental women dancer-choreographers—how they didn't and couldn't fit into older dance forms. Rainer tried, but was rejected (and ejected herself). I thought, How does a body move if it's not choreographed by others? My provisional answer was "breath and REM," which I imagined as both within "me" and inscribed by "your dream."

My next line responded to the way your line picked up on waking into movement. And I wanted to bring in those missed trees again. Dance and imagination compensating for what's been lost. The slash created even more "missing" between the words "missing" and "trees."

I was intrigued and perplexed by the question you posed, "is it / still / a story." One thing it suggested was, "What is dance now, when you don't have traditional narratives like, say, Swan Lake?"—in other words, the same question one might ask about any postmodern art form. My response, "*a no to virtuosity*," is a line from a manifesto Yvonne Rainer wrote. (The manifesto dogged her for decades, dance critics constantly referring to it, whereas she'd meant it provisionally, in relation to just one work.) The call and response about story and virtuosity could also be about our poem and our project.

I read your next line as an alternate proposition: "OK, I/we have said it's probably not a story, and no to virtuosity, so here's what I/we want." "Regard" means "see" and also connotes appreciating and caring for another being. But the line contains another layer of complexity: the I/we wants to be both visible and invisible. "Stripped/available" feels like a state that could be both highly visible and stripped of the visible (and goes back to the naked body I was imagining). The line is stripped, available—only two words to digest.

Your next line gets at a sense of vulnerability that echoes both the wanting and the being stripped, while segueing back to the trope of sleeping. Returning to the dream tattoo in the final line felt right given how far the poem travels between beginning and end.

It's warm and clear and sunny here. The stars were out in legions even above the city—Big Dipper! Little Dipper!

Regards,
Sarah

Dear Sarah,

For that first poem, I borrowed Simone Forti's reference to missing trees, seeing in it an opportunity to reflect on the vanishing ecosystem—a topic never far from my mind. At the same time, I wanted to engage with the notion of film, which made me think of photography—both the idea of visual images and an actual film negative, as well as negative space— another tie-in to those disappeared trees.

On a more personal level, I added a line about a "story," drawn from a training I attended a few years ago that addressed the stories we are told about ourselves when we are young. That I am unable to dance is a story I have told myself—and one that has had various implications in my life. Yet, despite my awareness of the dubious nature of such stories, I believe this is a truth about myself. (Does it still count as a "story" if it's true?)

Your reference to a dream tattoo felt particularly resonant for me; in other projects, I've explored the topic of skin—my own skin, as well as the evolution and anthropology of human skin—and the notion of invisibility, feeling unseen in various contexts. I've often felt conflicted between feeling ignored or dismissed, and wanting simply to blend in. Also, prior to starting this project, you and I had discussed the process of documenting dreams and incorporating that imagery and "experience" into our writing, so I found this reference in our collaboration especially fitting.

For me, the slash mark offers the option of keeping a thought open, allowing freedom to move to a related thought before the first is complete, and broader range of interpretation.

Ah, your description of the stars . . . I'm desperate for nicer weather—it's coming but slow . . . we are building a fire pit in our yard and I am excited to make use of it . . . after the rains!

With "we are advised to start fresh," did you have a particular theme in mind? I read "the grass is greener" as an expression of longing as well as a callout about climate, which seems a recurring theme in the project. Also, I interpreted "replace names with games / arrive at a practice" as, in part, a discussion of our process. I am curious as to how you came to that line, or perhaps more accurately, how it came to you.

Val

Dear Val,

Now I see the environmental issue embedded in "missing trees." I think that was there for me under the surface, as was the personal meaning of "story," now that you _____ that. ("Raise"? "articulate"? "surface"! That's the word I was looking for!)

Another thing I like about the slash is that it's what indicates a line break when a lineated poem is quoted in running text. So it's kind of an internal line break, and has some of the same powers of encouraging a _____ reading ("recursive"!) back and forth across the slash— whose other name, as you probably know, is "virgule."

What drew me to "we are advised to start fresh" is Stein's notion of beginning again and again, and the way that ties into the Buddhist concept of beginner's mind. It suggests this practice we've developed of creating a series of poems using one repeating procedure with new content in each iteration, and also what I think is required in life, a gazillion times per day—dropping all projections and thoughts of past and future and becoming a tabula rasa. John Cage (Merce Cunningham's partner) was Buddhist, and both of them influenced the choreographers we're befriending via this project (not to mention lots of other contemporary artists).

"The grass is greener when the sun is yellow" is a line Yvonne Rainer repeated in a dance she created. To me it suggests randomness and irreverence spliced with the discipline of a procedure—a combination often featured in her work. I employed it to reinforce and play with your previous line, "for one night try only to stand / each one / and I was in one of the boxes"—which evoked for me the discipline of procedure (while also connoting being "boxed" in a dismissive way). Similarly in "if I gave numbers to my motor centers" I was thinking about chance operations. (In the latter line I also felt it was important to address the disparity in standards for males and females in your line "if I wanted to play but boys never need to know how." To honor it, while providing a possible way forward.)

Curious how you're interacting with the Forti material, especially in light of the fact that dance has been a fraught topic for you. And can I say, how courageous of you to use this project as a way to investigate an area of _____ ("discomfort"? "challenge"? "trauma"?).

Yours,
Sarah

Dear Sarah,

I didn't know the other name for the slash. Ha, I just tried to type a period and accidentally typed a slash /

The gaps in your last letter leave a range of possible options for how to fill in the blanks. Or maybe you were interpreting what I had said but didn't want to misrepresent. But then it seems you selected the "right" word after some thought. So perhaps it also reveals your thought process, which I sense is largely the point.

I now recall that you mentioned Buddhism as a topic to explore in our project, and I see that the ideas of both Stein and Cage certainly fit with that mindset and with our work here. I heard recently that the average person has only about 4,500 days in which they can truly live (not be working, sleeping, etc.) (A subjective and flawed estimate.)

In a way, the line "we are about to start fresh" is a challenging one to follow—so open, no limits. What's your relationship to the use of constraints in your writing?

With this poem, I was thinking about kinesthetic intelligence ("*what I knew about things through my body*"), something my former taiko teacher, a trained dancer, would discuss when encouraging us to dance. I'm also playing with memories of experiences where dance was either mildly traumatic, as when I failed auditions because of the dance component, or the random mix of encounters—some dreadful, some sublime—at dance clubs. The "boys never need to know how" recalls my sense that expectations of men are different—specifically, my perception that boys didn't need to be able to dance to make the cut of a musical cast. This speaks to broader issues around double standards for men and women (a topic perhaps beyond the scope of this collaboration).

Thus far, I've focused on incorporating Forti's language into the poems through chance—yet I find myself resistant to giving over to true randomness, wanting to deliberately select lines to juxtapose with yours or adapt them to fit. I suppose I'll never be a true devotee of this practice! In reading her interviews, I've certainly come to appreciate her poetic use of language, which has provided endless opportunities for entering and extending our material. I'm also struck by the highly conceptual nature of her work.

"Virgule" comes from "little twig," diminutive of virga, "shoot, rod, stick."

I tried to write/save this on my phone on an interminable bus ride, but the changes were lost . . . ah, the perks/woes of technology.

Val

a stillness absorbing / awed murmurs of / milling day trippers

an arrangement of trees, let me count the rings

can you call a tree a body, body tree

when all that is left is fake nature

a ghostly structure, etched in the dawn

to understand fog or / *strategies of certain plants*

the landscape is a wild sister

I wanted to find something to climb

I felt like a cuckoo in a Swiss clock

sounding the passage of time

can you call a song prosthesis

substitute / what moves

I wrote an ear that composed all this

sogging the ground beneath our master plan

watch movements / not knowing whether rains or where

the future holds / the grade

what projections can be made when there are no more suns

when the heat emanates from

our gestures generative / between dark and light

moving / ribcages back and forth

reminiscent of breath

of wind of waves of fog rolling in

far from the equator / the edge divide daylight

we play languid in the sand

search idly for a patch of sun / can predictions be made when there
are no more stars

we wait our turn for the diagonal leap-run-run

<u>I am profoundly grateful for everything in my life</u>
<u>but at the same time, in a sour mood</u>

if I could define flexibility

feelings are facts / the mind is a muscle

because I have mass and I have weight / I can still feel gravity

rooted in space, so to speak, even while in motion

it doesn't get much better than this

handling / whiplash / combinations

feelings are arcs / let me trace the course

become a comet's tail

omen or ellipse / stream away

thru the paling night

a path known yet shaped by one small moon

like an unsaintly deity

like a polar bear swinging his head

Hi Val,

"Virgule" is from my copyediting past. The gaps represent all you suggest. Also, I was fatigued and trying to turn that into an asset.

4,500 days: the number presses. Can fear be a motivator? Or just drop all that and return to this moment.

To me, the line "we are advised to start fresh" does have a built-in constraint—the constraint of starting fresh. But I can see how it could feel too open. I'm always looking for that sweet spot between radically open and safely contained.

I'd like to know more about your fraught relationship to dance.

I don't mind double standards seeping in. Your approach to Forti's language sounds similar to the way I'm working with Rainer's. If I were to select phrases from the latter's work based wholly on chance, it wouldn't accord with the standards I'm attached to concerning what makes a poem "good" in terms of its music, imagery, meaning, and so forth. By the same token I'm leaning into chance in that I'm being led in fresh directions by phrases lifted from source texts.

Thank you for "little twig."

The political situation presses. I almost suggested that the poem "the system is a wild landscape" be about politics but it didn't feel right. I went with the theme of nature, which some of our other poems also address, like "we hope that the weather will continue." I'm waiting for a first line that lends itself to rolling in the smelly muck of politics. Regarding the poem "we hope . . ." I'm interested in how the theme of the destruction of nature gets superimposed with positive notions about presence, creativity, and a healthy loss of control. Speaking of which, what does this project do to the roles of writer and reader? To my mind it heightens that we are both both.

I picked up the little twig you sent and place it here, now, for you: /

Warm regards,
Sarah

Sarah,

I never learned the word "virgule" but everything I know about editing I learned in middle school. I like the idea of filling in gaps or having gaps to fill. As for my own story, there isn't much to say, I just could never dance. But my best friends growing up were dancers, and I always wondered what that meant.

I like the idea of a sweet spot.

Regarding constraints, a photographer I know, describing a project she did while traveling abroad, said something like, "Before arriving I learned that people here don't like being photographed. How can you create compelling imagery while still including an element of humanity? It's like solving a puzzle . . . and often you end up with better results than when you work without limits."

I wondered where "double standard" came from and discovered its relation to "single standard," which I'd never heard of. "The system only works when there's a single standard of conformity."

What is little twig? Oh, is that the virgule?

The notion of us as both reader and writer . . . a collective "I." Filtering and interpreting what we read/what is written, producing text to be filtered/interpreted . . . a system of creation and analysis. A collective eye.

Although you ultimately selected a different theme for the poem, I still sensed a political undercurrent in "the system is a wild landscape"— nature has become political too.

In thinking about "I am profoundly grateful . . ." what does it mean that when we acknowledge the simultaneity of gratitude and despair, we travel to space? What can we learn through the course of a small solar body?

—V

bound as two / the ropes are close enough

though our glissade-assemblé may be unpolished, we sure can leap

what's the difference between slide and glide

a gamut of moves from "dancey" to simple hauling of mattresses

such creative endeavors / keep us practiced at avoiding sleep

in this *saison* of our discontent we / *grapevine / moonwalk / time step*

we are thinking of a word like maneuvering

and putting *garlands of flowers on each bed*

heads pressed against each other yet / untroubled

even in *the throes of fighting for balance*

still thinking of the word / troubled

even as we *thunder clap / feather step / gancho*

we place our hands on the floor

<u>the next thought contains a note of defiance</u>

a refusal to spin and turn

catapults me into new terrain

make a fabric protect me, its frame of thin ribs

glazed in Mercury's dust

if airborne or dropped / forget to breathe

resist walking *through the eye of a needle*

proceed to sing the tone of a space

shimmy down it to the ground

on a leafless stem

breathe audibly, run out of breath, sweat

fresh water in, salt water out

of my realism

I come to call this / logomotion

V:

Speaking of gaps, the one between your discomfort with dance and your closeness to dancers feels fertile. As for me, early I found a home in dance. Socially awkward adolescent, yet when I danced I knew grace. But formal ballet and modern classes were traumatic—the standards for how to look and move felt unattainable. Later, I embraced modern— loving the combination of expression and rigour, and not caring as much if I excelled.

Lately, dance is too practical—wiggling in my living room to move my body per the daily quota. But yoga in a sweating group has new appeal (and it too is dancerly).

You chose dance language as the theme for the poem "we are using the word liaison." This poem felt so informed by that "we." I thought of this collaboration, and the way poetry can feel its way into any space, including a dance floor populated by leotarded bodies. I thought of Yvonne Rainer and the dancers who collaborated with her, and the endlessly innovative series of movements she has created, over decades.

Thank you for sharing the photographer's thoughts. Why shouldn't a valid constraint be respect for a people's way of being? As in, do not take my image—in this age of the image.

The word "system" has come up repeatedly in language you've contributed to this project. "The system is a wild landscape"; "the system only works when there's a single standard of conformity"; "a system of creation and processing." What draws you to this word?

Re: the poem starting "I am profoundly grateful . . ."—a comet flying through the air is a figure solitary yet sure.

Once I read a series of letters between Lyn Hejinian and Dodie Bellamy; Lyn (I think) wrote, Isn't it interesting how we letter writers tend to anchor ourselves in place and time? Dear Val, I write from the heart of Trump Country, where I'm doing a residency. The houses are small, the yards large. It snowed this morning, May 1st. Later I will walk on cold, flat streets, wave at strangers staring at me from trucks (they stare, yes, but they do wave back).

Yours,
Sarah

Dear Sarah,

Maybe one reason I've never gotten into yoga is that it is "dancerly," as you put it. I've always felt out of my element in that realm. They say no one is looking at you, but that isn't true—I would often be watching the others. I prefer Pilates because, to my mind, it focuses more on strength than grace.

With "we are using the word liaison," I was thinking about how the language of dance mirrors poetry. I tried to recall the terms I heard as a child, watching my best friend practice ballet.

Earlier this year, I watched *The OA*, which centers around a sequence of movements that open another dimension. This seemed remarkable, that dance could have such impact. Have you felt a sense of power through dance?

On a different note, the words "troubled" and "untroubled" in that poem remind me of the book *Troubling the Line*. What do you make of that word, "troubling"?

I am not sure where my fascination with systems originated, but I've been thinking about poetry in this way for some time. I suppose that this mindset first emerged when I was working at a computer science publisher and wrote a series of autobiographical poems using CS terminology; I used that "system" of language to process my own experiences. I often find that thinking about poetry in a systematic way can be helpful—perhaps as a way to avoid getting overly sentimental or "arty" in my writing.

We are corresponding from very different locales indeed—I in the Northwest (a reluctant transplant), in a house I call the cabin in the city. Spring has arrived. I've never lived anywhere so lush—I rely on friends to identify unfamiliar flowers and shrubs. I am hopeful that the snows have finally passed for the year.

Tell me about writing with "a note of defiance."

—V

V,

I tried Pilates once but due to injuries couldn't do many of the "core" (ha ha) moves without re-injuring. I envy Pilates aficionados—that balance, those rock-hard abs!

I haven't equated dance with power so much as with freedom. It can be a way to simultaneously express and lose the self. Some forms, such as Haitian dance, are designed to help the dancer move beyond what we might call the "small self" into the spiritual realm. In other forms, like contemporary dance, that's not necessarily the goal, but it happens anyway, at least for me. Imminence and transcendence, joined.

"Trouble" as a verb originates, so far as I know, in the King James Bible ("For an angel went down at a certain season into the pool, and troubled the water: whosoever then first after the troubling of the water stepped in was made whole of whatsoever disease he had." (John 5:3–4) Paul Simon's "Bridge Over Troubled Water" may be echoing that passage. Simon's "troubled" seems akin to "bothered," addressing a state of emotional upset that the speaker will soothe by "laying me down." More compelling for me is the use of the verb in the spiritual "Wade in the Water," in which it's God who's "gonna trouble the water." In that song, the passage I quoted mixes with other Biblical references to water, including the Jordan River and God's parting of the Red Sea, the latter especially pointing to liberation and justice. The tune and deliberate pace combine with the lyrics to create a powerful sense that justice will be served—God will trouble the waters in a way that will be very good for the righteous, and very ominous (troubling) for the bad (the troublesome).

The anthology *Troubling the Line* seems to echo this notion. I read "the line" as both the poetic line and the traditional lines we've drawn around gender. Steph Burt's review of the anthology equated "troubling" with "queering," "bending," and "breaking": "People who label themselves as genderqueer are trying to queer (or 'trouble,' or bend, or break) the binary of gender, to live as both/and or as neither/nor." (*Los Angeles Review of Books*, 11/17/13)

I like all of these slants on the verb "trouble" and the way they overlap. I like the idea of stepping into healing waters. I like the idea of bending and breaking rigid categories. I like the idea that justice will be served.

I want to know about "arty" and your resistance to it.

Re: "A note of defiance": I forgot which of us came up with that line. Had to reverse-engineer from a line I know I wrote—"glazed in Mercury's dust"—but part of me liked not knowing. That's a form of defiance that goes back at least as far as high school. I avoided memorizing my class schedule each quarter because—using a logic that now seems astonishingly self-defeating—I wanted to circumvent knowing what would happen in advance. Staying glazed seemed more free.

We transgress to gain freedom, no?

Yours,
S

the mind still at the departure gate

let ourselves be lulled

gaze at white blanketing a world

when bodies at wildly different speeds / this is turbulence

place the mask / breathe normally

reiterate phrases

the mind has yet to check in

and the black box pings

like in a *well-made horror movie called Can You Top This*

but I want to make the audience laugh

the most patriotic of acts

then an angel disappears out the window

the mind pondering what / to pack

<u>a mouse hurries across the space</u>

the idea of actualizing movement / what's the worst that could happen

fight, fly or freeze

mistaken as a still life

inside my shattered head

wrecked with waiting only to be cast / aside

dance of thumping heart, hunched shoulders, chattering knees

do not look just run out of the room screaming

like a *Freudian banshee*

does this mean I'm about to die

something I do every day

can recurrence keep me comfortable enough

is seriality the same as hanging off a cliff

a habit formed and fervently / followed

S—

Since moving to Portland, my partner and I have been taking Pilates classes regularly. Our teacher is extremely affirming—which I greatly appreciate! He's got a mellifluous voice—almost sings as he moves us from one pose to the next. I like the feeling of growing stronger and making consistent progress over time. I like being forced out of my head, to connect with my body.

When I said I resisted "arty," perhaps I was thinking about wanting to be taken seriously, and how if considered "arty," I might not be. This is making me think about process—one of my favorite writing topics. When I set out to draft this email, I made a brief outline in response to your points. As an editor, I am often parsing and analyzing tables of contents, and I've generally found that creating an outline can help focus and organize thoughts.

I was not aware of the derivation of "trouble"—or maybe I was once but have since forgotten. I have likely blocked out much of my Catholic upbringing. The word appears not just in pop and spirituals but in the blues and other genres. Its usage in lyrics is complex—its sound is pleasing but its meaning, of course, is not. Examining the word's origins, I've discovered its relationship to the word "turbulence," which appears in the sonnet "the plane has reached its cruising altitude." That poem seems to exude anxiety about current political realities.

Speaking of the phrase "troubling the line," which suggests a disruption to the norm or status quo, I'm also reminded of "Numbers Trouble" by Juliana Spahr and Stephanie Young (*Chicago Review*, 2007). This article challenges the notion that anthologies dedicated to writing by women (and more broadly, works addressing feminism in the experimental writing scene) are no longer necessary, because the publishing imbalance between men and women has been corrected over time. Given my experience working for a small press that publishes innovative writing by women, I, like the authors, am skeptical that this is the case. It seems noteworthy that the idea of "troubling" is so relevant in discussing the work of various marginalized communities.

Your question about transgression as freedom generates more questions. Are we, by virtue of our identity as experimental women writers, transgressive? Does the line at which a person/work/act is considered transgressive shift over time? Are we becoming more transgressive as a culture, or as "Numbers Trouble" suggests, are we in many ways stuck in a traditional society—still, in a sense, catching up?

Val

Val,

I like imagining your Pilates teacher singing you through movements.

Throughout this collaboration I've been observing the process leading up to the lines I contribute: the trajectory from wondering to considering to deciding to acting. When I first read your lines or proposed themes I often feel a bit stumped, simply because your contributions are the work of a mind not mine. Your own way of interpreting the previous line and responding to it, not to mention your music, imagery, and syntax, arrives in my inbox in a line like an exotic bird that I'm not sure how to care for. I have to think about how you might have arrived at that line based on the line I had sent you, and what meanings your line reinforces or proposes or makes possible. But then sometimes I find it easy to dance with your lines—for example, "a mouse hurries across the space."

Your use of an outline seems a perfect example of your love of structure, and a way to navigate the numerous topics this correspondence is generating. I find myself constantly wondering which threads to pick up, how much detail to provide, how much personal data relative to poetics (or is the personal data part of the poetics) . . . .

I looked up "arty." It does indeed have negative connotations: "showily or pretentiously artistic." I'm curious about the guidelines we set for ourselves as artists—where they come from, what they enable and disallow.

I do think "experimental" by definition means "transgressive." Looking back, it seems clear that the line whereby someone or something becomes transgressive shifts over time. Think of H.D., or Stein, or any artist whose work challenged the status quo—as their ideas seeped into art practices of others, and into the cultural consciousness, something different was then required to "Make It New!" (Pound). Yet has our society become more transgressive, even though it has made room (in a limited way) for innovative art? That's a hard one. Experimental art is up against incredibly sophisticated forces of commercialism and exploitation, which I think of as the very opposite of healthy transgression. Spahr and Young's article rightly points to the need to be vigilant. But maybe my cynicism is a habituated response that keeps me from missing ways our culture truly has allowed more transgression.

—S

Sarah—

The line "a mouse hurries across the space" called to mind a recent experience I had at a reading where a rat fell on the man behind me and mayhem ensued. I chose the theme of irrational fear in response (I did, in fact, scream and listen to the rest of the reading from outside the room). Perhaps the reason this one felt so intuitive is that fear is such an accessible emotion that the lines sort of just tumbled out of us.

Reflecting further on "art" and its derivations ... "art," "arty," "artifice"... I am struck by the often negative connotations of these terms. "Artifice" means a trick, a cunning or crafty device. Interesting that the earlier meaning (circa 1530s) was workmanship, or something made with craft or skill. The modern meaning came about in the 1650s. What does it say that over time, these words have taken on a more negative meaning? Has "art" itself been devalued over time?

In human culture, I wonder if transgression, like progress, swings like a pendulum. You and I likely have more freedom than our predecessors; there is more innovative art, greater inclusion of artists/authors of different backgrounds and identities than ever. And yet. Perhaps because of this newfound openness, the traditional forces push back. This seems most evident in political spheres, at this moment. For example: the prevalence of views such as those on the "alt right," which previously would have been considered unacceptable in public discourse. There is a strange and frightening resistance to "the Other" because those historically in power no longer have full control. Meanwhile, artists are playing a key role in the resistance against these "traditional" forces. Which I think supports your point that experimentation is, by definition, transgressive.

As our last few sonnets approach completion, I'm especially curious to hear about your chosen theme for the poem "I begin to arrange"— spontaneity. An apt descriptor for this project as a whole.

—V

I begin to arrange

unscripted remarks and laughter

objects in space *(interweave flickering)*

at my body's house

like birds in a flight cage

redefine territory

the difference between inhabit and invasion

the best solution

improvised wings

turn us loose

inside our enclosures

the light from our eyes

illuminating our mind's I

preparing us for what

we lie under boxes / whistle

what "going away" signifies

reflect / like a pool

accumulate / tiny bits of movement

deep feelers / are we really down here

no history no / tears

the name in the negative

slows our sounds and sentences

the pattern fractured / bones

in our *mannequin dance*

and at the end we see it all

we turn our *butterflies loose*

edgewise to the sun

V,

In this process of creating poems that complicate the notion of the separate self, I've been feeling a visceral sense of the "I" ballooning to include the "we." And then I wonder, is it that the self is expanding, or am I merely remembering what's always been true, that the one contains the many?

Leslie Scalapino often avoided the pronoun "I," using "one" instead. I admit I once judged this gesture as precious or forced. I've reflected a lot since then about her motivations. Was she determined to take a stand by using language that reflected as accurately as possible the truth as she viewed it? Or did she use "one" as a practice, to train herself to align with an understanding of reality that all too easily slips away in quotidian life and speech? I don't know for sure but more and more I draw (one draws) inspiration from her habit.

You asked for my thoughts about the theme of spontaneity for the poem "I begin to arrange." That phrase reminded me of the ways we try to control our art and our lives, which brought up the opposite—the spontaneity we've employed in this project. And of course even when one has anticipated spontaneity, it doesn't necessarily arrive the way one had intended. One "begins to arrange" and then all hell breaks loose. One can fight that, or relax into it.

Maybe someone knows the answer for why the valence of "artifice" has shifted over time, from craft to crafty. The story of Western society is one of ever greater splintering of community until each individual is either metaphorically or literally a businessperson, hawking whatever we've got to everyone else. Being on the make requires craftiness as much as, or more than, craft. Speaking of transgression in art, I worry that what I see as the art world's healthy resistance to the status quo is getting more polluted over time by the materialism and pressure to "make it" prevalent in society at large. I want to believe in the pendulum theory, and do see the shorter-term swings you describe. I write this fresh on the heels of Robert Mueller's appointment as special counsel for the Russia debacle. Will justice be served?

Our last two sonnets feel both aerated and embodied to me. I'm wondering if that's because at this point we've developed our chops more. I also notice the lines tend to be a little shorter in these poems. Maybe that makes it easier to swing with them?

I'm sad this project is drawing to a close. And curious to see how it ripples out into whatever happens next—for "me," for "you," for "us"—for anybody.

Warm regards,
S

May 20

Dear Sarah,

I think you're back in San Francisco now. This project itself has been a journey, one in many ways rooted in the Bay Area—where we met and where you still reside. Over the course of the project, we have both traveled to/from there, and many of the writers and work we have drawn from originated there. Surely the aesthetics and philosophies prevalent in that area have informed both of our writing practices, and by extension, this project.

I think a lot more about location and the implications of living in and traveling into different landscapes now that I live in Portland, which I've discovered is a much wilder landscape than anywhere I've previously lived. I continually observe my garden with awe, as countless flowers, trees, and shrubs (most planted prior to my arrival and still unidentified by me) sprout and radically alter the space, every day. My mother is visiting in four days, and I am crossing my fingers that the irises (one of the few plants I recognize) are still in bloom! Thinking about these crossovers and observations of space and locale, I wanted to bring in some of what I've now learned about Simone Forti. One obvious connection is that, among other places she has lived, she attended Reed College, just a couple miles south of here; she then moved to San Francisco for a time. These kinds of overlaps between us and the artists we have invited into the project feel natural, almost a given at this point.

Beyond these geographical overlaps, delving more deeply into her work… of all the pieces I read about, the one I found most affecting and relevant to our project is *Sleep Walkers/Zoo Mantras*. This piece was inspired by her observations of zoo animals—specifically wild animals genetically predisposed to travel great distances—whose repetitive movements in confinement are driven by boredom and a need to comfort themselves. Forti wrote: "In every bear, gorilla, or person, there's an ability to retain the essence of one's nature regardless of how much the pattern of one's life system has been fractured or taken away."

It's heartbreaking to contemplate the reality of zoo animals that Forti conveys. Also, this example offers another lens through which to explore the question of identity. I saw here a way of relating animals to people (or all creatures to each other) as well as underscoring how in the most fundamental way we are all essentially the same. A gorilla is a gorilla, a bear is a bear, a person is a person no matter how our environment changes, or how our culture emphasizes difference. (This also echoes your thoughts in the last letter about the "I" ballooning to "we," of one containing many.) On a personal level, I want to maintain my San Francisco self even though I am living in a new environment. Like you, I want to see justice served, for all to be treated fairly and equally. And also: if all members of a species are of the same nature, then I am you, you are me, we are we, I is we.

Regarding the last two poems in the series, our notion of them being easier to "swing with" echoes the way Forti spoke of animal movements, the way a polar bear swings its head.

It feels strange that our collaboration is drawing to a close. But for the last poem you chose the line "the site of an eternal performance," which suggests that maybe this conversation will continue in some way.

I wanted to end the poem with a particular line, and I tried to build in lines that would lead up to it. But my attempt was predictably thwarted by the nature of collaboration. In your last line, you wrote "we turn our *butterflies loose*" so it seemed too unwieldy to introduce another creature. But thinking of a line from earlier in the poem, "*reflect / like a pool*," I added as my penultimate line "and at the end we see it all." And the line I had considered closing with, the name of one of Forti's works, was *Turtles All the Way Down in the Water*.

Yours,
Val

NOTES

Some of the language in this book has been adapted from the following sources:

Boynton, Andrew. "No Mistakes: Simone Forti." *The New Yorker* (November 2012). www.newyorker.com/culture/culture-desk/no-mistakes-simone-forti

Lim, Nancy. "MoMA Collects: Simone Forti's *Dance Constructions*." *INSIDE/OUT* (January 2016). www.moma.org/explore/inside_out/2016/01/27/moma-collects-simone-fortis-dance-constructions

Newton, Michael and Russo, Emmalea. *Eternal Apprentice*. Minneapolis: Double Cross Press. 2016.

Picard, Caroline. "The Sensation of Un-thought Thoughts: An Interview with Simone Forti." *Art21 Magazine* (April 2016). http://magazine.art21.org/2016/03/01/the-sensation-of-un-thought-thoughts-an-interview-with-simone-forti

Rainer, Yvonne. *Feelings Are Facts: A Life*. Cambridge, MA: MIT Press Writing Art series. Edited by Roger Conover. 2006.

Schlenzka, Jenny. "Simone Forti: Drunk with Movement." *Flash Art* (November–December 2009). www.flashartonline.com/article/simone-forti

Wikipedia. "Simone Forti." https://en.wikipedia.org/wiki/Simone_Forti

Wikipedia. "Yvonne Rainer." https://en.wikipedia.org/wiki/Yvonne_Rainer

AFTER-WORDS

Greetings! Thank you both for talking to us about your process today!
Can you introduce yourselves, in a way that you would choose?

VW: I'm interested in the intersection of words and other media, such as visual art, music, and technology; *Blade Runner*-esque explorations of relationships (with baseball references inserted, as needed); and collaborative projects related to origami flower-folding, reclaiming language related to restricting of women's rights, and now, the works of postmodern dancers.

With Chicago-based artist Jennifer Yorke, I've developed projects based on my manuscripts 'Flood Diary' and 'A Rupture in the Interiors,' which culminated in exhibitions in Berkeley and Chicago, as well as a residency in La Porte Peinte in Noyers, France. I'm a co-founder of the Bay Area Correspondence School, where I've exchanged mail art; spearheaded the writing of a collaborative Facebook poem about the "war on women," which led to the creation of the chapbook *A Body You Shall Be*; and helped coordinate multiple events, most notably the BACS Variety Show and Art Extravaganza in 2017. For eight years I was a member of Kelsey Street Press, a long-standing publisher of innovative writing by women.

My first book, *a game of correspondence*, was published by Black Radish Books in 2015, and my chapbooks include *It's been a long time since I've dreamt of someone* (Dancing Girl Press) and *The history of mining* (ge collective/Poetry Flash).

A native St. Louisan, I arrived in San Francisco in 2003 and lived in the Bay Area for 12 years; I currently reside up the road in Portland, OR. I received my MFA in Writing from the University of San Francisco. In my daytime hours, I edit education books in Portland. More at valeriewitte.com

SRR: My work charts the space between limitation and freedom. It documents ways we can be trapped by socially imposed rules of any kind. My writing also explores how repressive childhood experiences and a variety of traumas can calcify into debilitating beliefs and habits. At the same time, it asserts the right to take up space, take risks, liberate self and word and form. It enacts these freedoms by foregrounding creative process, including the creative potential of error, damage, and fragments; by addressing taboo subjects; by using surreal/dream imagery and linguistic structures that defy reason; and by dissolving boundaries between inner and outer, self and other. My projects have tended to focus on female characters who are identifiable and porous/multiple. I employ creative processes that ensure the work generated will surprise and teach me.

My poetry collection *Lizard* blends aspects of contemporary womanhood with facts about various lizard species to question what it means to be a human at this historical moment, in relation to other humans, other species, and the planet. My book *Manhatten* combines fiction, lineated poems, dream matter, and art reviews to tell the story of a young woman coming of age in New York City. A narrator named Sarah Rosenthal, who may or may not be the author, navigates experiences and relationships that are by turns disturbing and comical, in prose that borrows much from poetry including associative leaps across time and space, and pleasure in language's musicality. Other publications include the chapbooks *The Animal* (a collaboration with visual artist Amy Fung-yi Lee), *not-chicago*, *sitings*, and *How I Wrote This Story*. I am the editor of *A Community Writing Itself: Conversations with Vanguard Writers of the Bay Area*.

Besides the collaboration mentioned above and my collaboration with Valerie Witte focusing on postmodern dance, I was a founding member of diSh, a performance ensemble that created pieces combining words and gestures, and am currently working with multimedia poet and translator Denise Newman on creating a platform featuring reviews of underrepresented literature by individuals who have limited or no prior experience reading or responding to such texts. I live in San Francisco where I am a jurist for the California Book Awards and a Life and Professional Coach. I also develop language arts curricula for the Center for the Collaborative Classroom. More at sarahrosenthal.net.

Why are you a poet/writer/artist?

VW: My primary reason for being an artist/writer is to build and be part of community—a community that appreciates and makes work that can be any or all of the following: thought-provoking, innovative, playful, entertaining, engaging, inspiring. And by community, I mean: if I can reach at least one other person through my work, I feel fulfilled. I can hardly remember a time when I wasn't writing. It is something I have been doing since I knew how, what I've dedicated more time and effort to than anything else. I'm generally happiest when I'm writing. It's what brings meaning to my life, for which I am very grateful.

SRR: I create because I revel in the human imagination, an astounding capacity of our species and one that provides enormous joy and meaning, especially for the maker. I create because I see it as my best shot at contributing in a worthwhile way to the polis. Making art is both the easiest and the hardest thing that I do. I don't feel fully alive when I'm not doing it.

When did you decide you were a poet/writer/artist (and/or: do you feel comfortable calling yourself a poet/writer/artist? and/or: what other titles or affiliations do you prefer/feel are more accurate)?

VW: I've been writing since I was a young child, so I've been comfortable with the term poet/writer for a long time. I don't recall a specific moment at which I began identifying as a poet/writer, but perhaps after I earned my MFA, or when I started publishing my work in literary journals—and certainly when I published my full-length book. I usually introduce myself as a book editor first and a poet second. These days people have such a strong reaction to the book editor ID (so many questions!) that I don't even get to "poet."

SRR: When I was three, I announced that I wanted to be an artist. I grew up in an art-appreciating home and loved trancing out by looking at the images of art on our walls. Being the person who made those objects seemed like the coolest vocation. The impulse to "be an artist" translated soon into creative writing, for which I had a natural affinity. I wrote as a child and teen and then lost touch with the impulse until a couple years out of college. When I rediscovered writing in my mid-twenties, it was like coming home. Since then I've described myself as primarily a poet, although I also write prose and enjoy engaging in other art forms including performance and visual art.

What's a "poet" (or "writer" or "artist") anyway?

VW: I view the term "artist" very broadly, as anyone who creates something new and innovative, especially if they are willing to share that creation with others. And perhaps, someone who sees beyond the literal, offering interpretations that involve a deeper level of nuance and thought, and moving others to see things in a different way.

SRR: Poets, artists traffic in visions, the visionary. They are comfortable swimming in dream realms where light and darkness intermix in surprising ways, and they work to translate their knowledge of these realms into art that helps others enter them as well. Poets, artists often find themselves on the outside looking into society's house. This is thanks to several complex variables including the fact that our society often looks askance at work that does not necessarily aim at accruing wealth, and the fact that by temperament artists often feel more comfortable moving between worlds, Hermes-like. Artists' marginal position often gives them empathy for others who find themselves positioned as outsiders.

What do you see as your cultural and social role (in the literary/artistic/creative community and beyond)?

VW: With my own art, I strive to engage people intellectually and encourage them to see things in new ways. But beyond my own work, I view my role within the poetry and broader art community as, chiefly, to help circulate the work; to that end, I have participated in several literary organizations on a voluntary basis, helping to produce and promote books and art, and collaborating with other artists and writers on projects and events. Especially right now, in the current political climate (and given the rising temperature of our planet's actual climate), I feel that art/poetry is one of the few realms that can truly offer hope, a way to open people's minds and make visible truths that perhaps cannot be seen as readily through other media (news, etc.). As part of this mindset, I've become more and more convinced that education is key; I've had the privilege of working professionally as an editor in educational book publishing for virtually my entire career, and I am also currently a board member of a literacy organization called First Book, which provides books to children in disadvantaged communities. Through these activities, I hope to contribute by delivering tools and resources to help people develop the literacy and critical thinking skills needed to participate fully in our culture--in the arts and beyond.

SRR: I think of myself as a participant in dialogue, which means it's incumbent upon me not only to express myself but to listen deeply. In terms of a poethics, I privilege the latter. Good listening is in short supply in our world, yet it's desperately needed. So regardless of which specific hat I'm wearing--poet, colleague, educator, curriculum designer, coach, editor, beloved--I try to show up open to what I'm hearing, ready to mirror it and to express my honest and caring response. At the least I can continually work on my capacity to provide this; at the most I can inspire others in the same direction.

I'm increasingly interested in what Harrell Fletcher refers to as social practice and relational aesthetics, an interest that my investigation of Yvonne Rainer's work has further nurtured. I am drawn to this approach to art-making for its potential to allow me to wear all or at least many of the above-mentioned hats simultaneously, and to activate inclusive projects and processes that encourage creative, attentive interaction among diverse participants.

Talk about the process or instinct to move these poems (or your work in general) as independent entities into a body of work. How and why did this happen? Have you had this intention for a while? What encouraged and/or confounded this (or a book, in general) coming together? Was it a struggle?

As we explain in the Poets' Note, we launched our collaboration by reading and discussing *Eternal Apprentice*, a chapbook by Michael Newton and

Emmalea Russo. As part of their discussion, they engage with John Cage and Merce Cunningham's ideas about chance operations, and we became interested in using the chapbook as source text as well as in employing random procedures in our project.

We noted Cunningham's role as a key figure in the evolution of contemporary dance, influencing several female choreographers who made significant contributions to the field. We also discovered that the two of us had radically different feelings about dance: Sarah has a mostly positive relationship to the form, whereas dance has more troublesome associations for Valerie. With all this in mind, we decided to each "adopt" a contemporary female dancer-choreographer who had worked at some point with Cunningham and Cage, letting our contributions be informed and inspired by these innovative women's lives and ideas, and thinking through our own respective relationships to dance. Valerie chose Simone Forti and Sarah chose Yvonne Rainer.

In developing this project's contours, we relied on our curiosity and a desire to take creative risks. Yet looking back, we recognize the shared feminist tenets that undergird this work. Collaborating on the poems challenges the traditional Western concept of the text written by a solo (male) author. The epistolary component adds embodiment to a project highly mediated by technology. In the letters we "show our hand" to one another and to the reader, creating a space of intimacy and vulnerability. Yet we strive to do so in a way that opens up, rather than forecloses, multiple readings of the poems. Each of us, and by extension our readers, are invited to "talk back" and bring other perspectives to the exchange.

What formal structures or other constrictive practices (if any) do you use in the creation of your work? Have certain teachers or instructive environments, or readings/writings/work of other creative people informed the way you work/ write?

VW: Structure almost always plays a key role in my work, and I typically use or create a different structure for every project. Examples include emails with subject lines and status updates, prose blocks that become more diffuse as a book unfolds, copious use of fragments spanning the entirety of a page. Constraints or conventions that serve to help me build these structures include consistent/nonstandard punctuation or capitalization, limiting the number of lines per poem, randomly selecting a number of "chapters" or pages in a section, and visual and verbal/written cues that indicate when a manuscript is looping and perhaps can be read in a different order or way, outside of linear time. I view my poems as building blocks which I ultimately assemble to create a coherent whole. Sometimes I start with a particular structure, adjusting it several times as I continue writing, until I feel that it truly fits the project.

My experience in the MFA program at USF was extremely influential. Before that time, my writing wasn't experimental at all. In fact I was resistant to experimental poetics, and I would absolutely not be writing the way I write if I hadn't attended this program. I found myself greatly inspired by my three classmates, Craig Santos Perez, Alexandra Mattraw, and Rebecca Stoddard; their work is always exciting, innovative, deeply original. I was similarly influenced by my teachers (and the writers they taught), such as Rusty Morrison and Susan Gevirtz, who introduced me to the writing of Barbara Guest. I was exposed again to Guest and many other influences later through my work with Kelsey Street Press, including Elizabeth Robinson and Bhanu Kapil. All of these writers push the boundaries of what poetry is or can be, which is what I also strive to do in my work.

SRR: The primary structure I work inside is the long form. I tend to take on a single larger topic and explore it for the length of a book or chapbook. This allows for a depth of engagement and a sense of being held within the contours of a project for a length of time. Each subject matter seems to require its own unique structure. For example, *Manhatten* comprises prose-poem-like columns interspersed with lineated poems. In *Lizard*, narrow, lineated poems, mostly a page or less in length, predominate. My manuscript 'Estelle Meaning Star' features cut-ups sourced from journal entries.

I was introduced to the long form as an MFA student at San Francisco State University, where many of the texts I encountered were book-length or longer (think of Robert Duncan, who envisioned his entire oeuvre as part of one ongoing book). Mentor texts from that period––far too many to name–– include works by Bernadette Mayer, Harryette Mullen, Eileen Myles, Theresa Hak-Kyung Cha, Leslie Scalapino, Lyn Hejinian, Barbara Guest, Edmond Jabès, and Kamau Braithwaite. Faculty I studied with included Myung Mi Kim, Aaron Shurin, Robert Glück, Norma Cole, and guest instructors Kathleen Fraser and Michael Palmer. The work of peers I encountered in the MFA program as well as in the larger Bay Area scene––most of whom were also working in the long form––also inspired me. Again the list is long but includes Dana Teen Lomax, Jennifer Firestone, Erin Wilson, Elise Ficarra, Stefani Barber, Sarah Anne Cox, Pamela Lu, and Aja Couchois Duncan.

Speaking of monikers, what does your title represent? How was it generated? Talk about the way you titled the book, and how your process of naming (individual pieces, sections, etc) influences you and/or colors your work specifically.

"The grass is greener when the sun is yellow" is a sentence that Yvonne

Rainer spoke in a section of her piece *Three Satie Spoons*. It appears as one of the lines in our book. We selected it as a title for its imagistic vividness as well as for the way it invites the reader to ponder and question. It proposes a relationship of juxtaposition––two separate things happening at the same time––while it simultaneously suggests cause and effect (sunshine is a factor supporting the growth of healthy grass). This vividness and multivalence hint at the lively engagement the book's contents encourage.

This sentence is the first instance of speech used by Rainer in her choreography. Incorporating speech was a practice she had learned from John Cage; it was also employed by Forti and other colleagues. In *Three Satie Spoons*, it works with gestures in a paratactic relationship, suggesting a rich, open-ended correspondence between language and dance, a correspondence fundamental to our project. Parataxis and collage are important elements to both of us as individual artists, so it's natural that we would draw on them as collaborators. They allow for a nonhierarchical interrelationship of diverse materials and ideas, one that invites readers to participate in the making of meaning.

What does this particular work represent to you as indicative of your method/ creative practice, your history, mission/intentions/hopes/plans?

Both of us bring to this work an intense personal relationship to dance and a fascination with the history of dance, in particular the postmodern era of Forti, Rainer, and their contemporaries. We share a love of epistolary form and of collaborative practice. The making of this book has spawned a longer project; we are now working on a collection of essays engaging our personal memories of dance and the work of Rainer and Forti. We hope, among other things, that *The Grass Is Greener When the Sun Is Yellow* as well as the larger project it has generated will bring the work of these choreographers and their colleagues to readers' attention, so that it can enrich others' lives as much as it has ours.

What does this book DO (as much as what it says or contains)?

This book enacts a dialogue between two writers who seek to understand the thinking behind the work of the artists they explore, and in the process, gain understanding of each others' experiences and process as well. It creates a space that is both welcoming and challenging, inviting readers to participate in the dialogue while making clear that the relationships between the authors, artists, and topics are layered and complex.

What would be the best possible outcome for this book? What might it do in the world, and how will its presence as an object facilitate your creative role in your community and beyond? What are your hopes for this book, and for your practice?

We hope the book will encourage readers to engage in multiple forms of conversation, not only inviting them to explore the work of Rainer, Forti, and other postmodern artists, but also inspiring them to generate their own discussions about their work and that of the art and artists that move them. This project has strengthened our capacity to engage in caring, egalitarian collaboration, and we hope the book as an object in the world will provide us with an entry point to present collaboration as a way of making art and a way of being in the world, and to support others who want help using it. We will continue the conversation we started in the manuscript through the essay project we are now working on.

Let's talk a little bit about the role of poetics and creative community in social and political activism, so present in our daily lives as we face the often sobering, sometimes dangerous realities of the Capitalocene. How does your process, practice, or work otherwise interface with these conditions? I'd be curious to hear some of your thoughts on the challenges we face in speaking and publishing across lines of race, age, ability, class, privilege, social/cultural background, gender, sexuality (and other identifiers) within the community as well as creating and maintaining safe spaces, vs. the dangers of remaining and producing in isolated "silos" and/or disciplinary and/or institutional bounds?

In the Age of the Orange Man we are called, more urgently than ever, to speak truth to power and stand against division. Artists and collectivities need to apply their creativity to generating innovative strategies to promote equity and healing, and refrain from causing further harm to our frayed polis, while generously sharing those strategies with others. This endeavor includes acknowledging our own blind spots and continuing to sensitize ourselves to multiple perspectives, taking up lines of investigation within our art that support minoritized groups, and creating or participating in frameworks, such as The Operating System, that take an explicitly activist, inclusive approach to disseminating poetry.

PROJECT COLLABORATORS

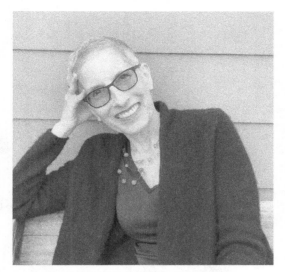

SARAH ROSENTHAL

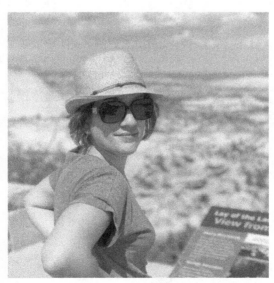

VALERIE WITTE

ABOUT THE COVER ART:

The Operating System 2019 chapbooks, in both digital and print, feature art from Heidi Reszies. The work is from a series entitled "Collected Objects & the Dead Birds I Did Not Carry Home," which are mixed media collages with encaustic on 8 x 8 wood panel, made in 2018.

Heidi writes: "This series explores objects/fragments of material culture—how objects occupy space, and my relationship to them or to their absence."

ABOUT THE ARTIST:

Heidi Reszies is a poet/transdisciplinary artist living in Richmond, Virginia. Her visual art is included in the National Museum of Women in the Arts CLARA Database of Women Artists. She teaches letterpress printing at the Virginia Commonwealth University School of the Arts, and is the creator/curator of Artifact Press. Her poetry collection titled *Illusory Borders* is forthcoming from The Operating System in 2019, and now available for pre-order. Her collection titled *Of Water & Other Soft Constructions* was selected by Samiya Bashir as the winner of the Anhinga Press 2018 Robert Dana Prize for Poetry (forthcoming in 2019).

Find her at heidireszies.com

WHY PRINT:DOCUMENT?
(AND WHAT DOES THIS MEAN FOR DIGITAL MEDIA?)

The Operating System has traditionally used the language "print:document" to differentiate from the book-object as part of our mission to distinguish the act of documentation-in-book-FORM from the act of publishing as a backwards-facing replication of the book's agentive *role* as it may have appeared the last several centuries of its history. Ultimately, we approach the book as TECHNOLOGY: one of a variety of documents across a range of media that humans have invented and in turn used to archive and disseminate ideas, beliefs, stories, and other evidence of production.

Ownership and use of printing presses and access to (or restriction of) information/materials, libraries, and archives has long been a site of struggle, related in many ways to revolutionary activity and the fight for civil rights and free speech all over the world. While (in many countries) the contemporary quotidian landscape has indeed drastically shifted in its access to platforms for sharing information and in the widespread ability to "publish" digitally, even with extremely limited resources, the importance of publication on physical media has not diminished. In fact, this may be the most critical time in recent history for activist groups, artists, and others to insist upon learning, establishing, and encouraging personal and community documentation practices.

With The OS's print endeavors I wanted to open up a conversation about this: the ultimately radical, transgressive act of creating PRINT / DOCUMENTATION in the digital age. It's a question of the archive, and of history: who gets to tell the story, and what evidence of our lives, our behaviors, and/or our experiences are we leaving behind? We can know little to nothing about the future into which we're leaving an unprecedentedly digital document trail—but we can be assured that publications, government agencies, museums, schools, and other institutional powers that be will continue to leave BOTH a digital and print version of their production for the official record. Will we?

As a (rogue) anthropologist and scholar, I can easily pull up many accounts about how lives, behaviors, experiences—how THE STORY of a time or place--was pieced together using the deep study of the archive: correspondence, notebooks, and other physical documents which are no longer the norm in many lives and practices. As we move our creative behaviors towards digital note taking, and even audio and video, what can we predict about future technology that is in any way assuring that our stories will be accurately told—or told at all? How will we leave these things for the record?

For all our years of print publication, I've said that "with these documents we say: WE WERE HERE, WE EXISTED, WE HAVE A DIFFERENT STORY," but now, with the rapid expansion of greater volume with digital and DIY printed media, we add: we ARE here, and while we are, we will not be limited in what we add value to, share, make accessible, or give voice to, by restricting it to what we can afford to print in volume.

Adding a digital series is the next chapter of *our* story: a way for us to support more creative practitioners and offer folks independent options for POD or DIY-zine-style distribution, even without our financial means changing—which means, each book will *also* have archive-ready print manifestations. It's our way of challenging what is required to evolve and grow. Ever onward, outward, beyond.

Elæ [Lynne DeSilva-Johnson]. Founder& Creative Director
THE OPERATING SYSTEM, Brooklyn NY 2019

THE 2019 OS CHAPBOOK SERIES

DIGITAL TITLES:

***

PRINT TITLES:

***

PLEASE SEE OUR FULL CATALOG
FOR FULL-LENGTH VOLUMES AND PREVIOUS CHAPBOOK SERIES:
HTTPS://SQUAREUP.COM/STORE/THE-OPERATING-SYSTEM/

DOC U MENT
/däkyəmənt/

First meant "instruction" or "evidence," whether written or not.

noun - a piece of written, printed, or electronic matter that provides information or evidence or that serves as an official record
verb - record (something) in written, photographic, or other form
synonyms - paper - deed - record - writing - act - instrument

[*Middle English, precept, from Old French, from Latin documentum, example, proof, from docre, to teach; see dek- in Indo-European roots.*]

Who is responsible for the manufacture of value?

Based on what supercilious ontology have we landed in a space where we vie against other creative people in vain pursuit of the fleeting credibilities of the scarcity economy, rather than freely collaborating and sharing openly with each other in ecstatic celebration of MAKING?

While we understand and acknowledge the economic pressures and fear-mongering that threatens to dominate and crush the creative impulse, we also believe that ***now more than ever we have the tools to relinquish agency via cooperative means,*** fueled by the fires of the Open Source Movement.

Looking out across the invisible vistas of that rhizomatic parallel country we can begin to see our community beyond constraints, in the place where intention meets resilient, proactive, collaborative organization.

Here is a document born of that belief, sown purely of imagination and will. When we document we assert. We print to make real, to reify our being there. When we do so with mindful intention to address our process, to open our work to others, to create beauty in words in space, to respect and acknowledge the strength of the page we now hold physical, a thing in our hand… we remind ourselves that, like Dorothy: *we had the power all along, my dears.*

THE PRINT! DOCUMENT SERIES
is a project of
the trouble with bartleby
in collaboration with
the operating system

Printed in the USA
CPSIA information can be obtained
at www.ICGtesting.com
LVHW091930280923
759620LV00007B/200